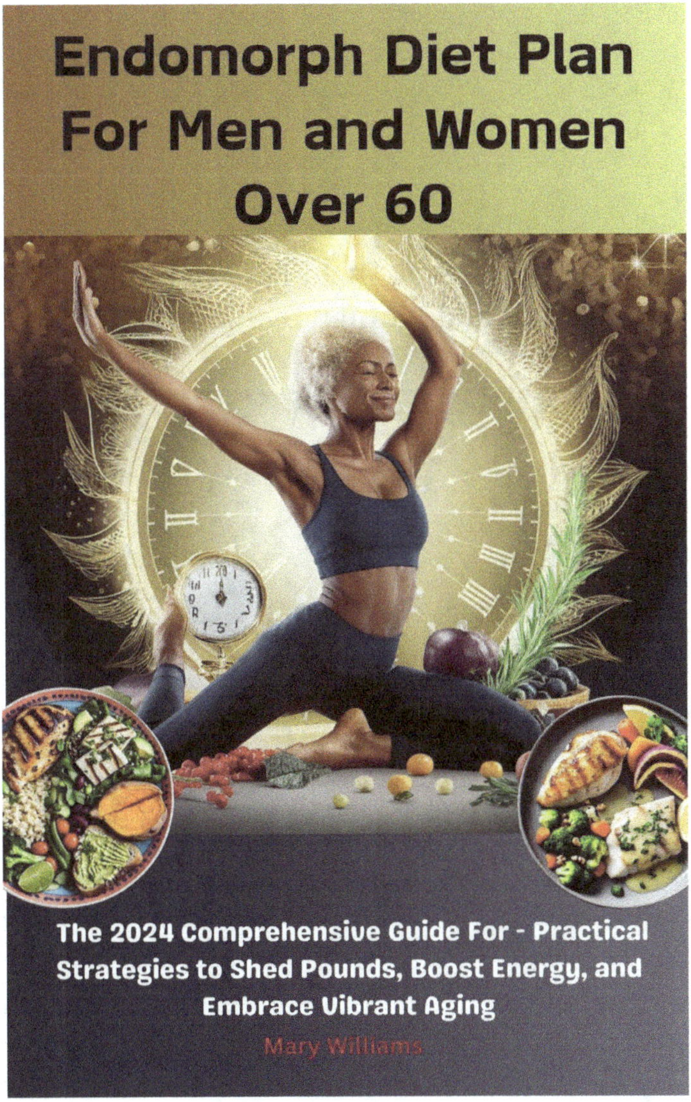

Endomorph Diet Plan For Men and Women Over 60

The 2024 Comprehensive Guide For - Practical Strategies to Shed Pounds, Boost Energy, and Embrace Vibrant Aging

Mary Williams

2

Endomorph Diet Plan For Men and Women Over 60

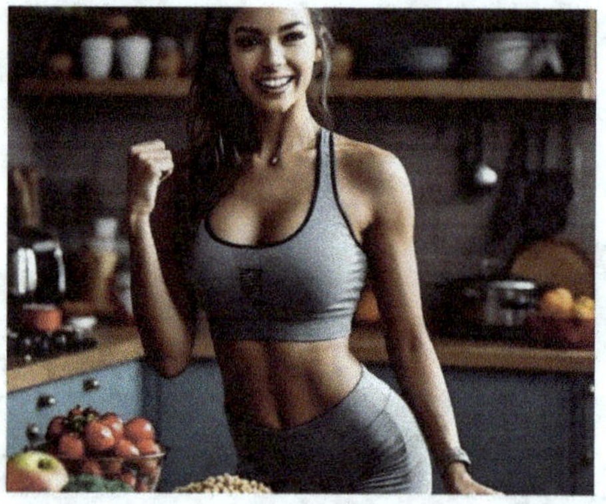

The Comprehensive Guide For – Practical Strategies to Shed Pounds, Boost Energy, and Embrace Vibrant Aging

3

4

<u>GRATITUDE SPEECH</u>

Good day ladies and gentlemen,

I want to begin by expressing my deepest gratitude to each and every one of you for being here today. Your support and participation in this event means so much.

Most importantly, I want to thank you all for purchasing my book. As an author, seeing people enjoy my work and find value in the messages and stories I've shared is incredibly rewarding. It truly would not have been possible without readers like yourself who are willing to give a newcomer such as myself a chance.

I have put my heart and soul into writing this book in the hopes that it could help or inspire others in some way. That it has connected with you is more than I could have asked for. You have not only supported my dream of being a published author, but you have helped this book reach new audiences so that it can make a bigger impact. For that, I am eternally grateful.

This is just the beginning of my journey, and I hope you will continue following along to see where the story goes next. Thank you again for your interest, investment and for helping make my vision a reality. I appreciate each and every one of you more than I can say. Thank you and enjoy the rest of your day!

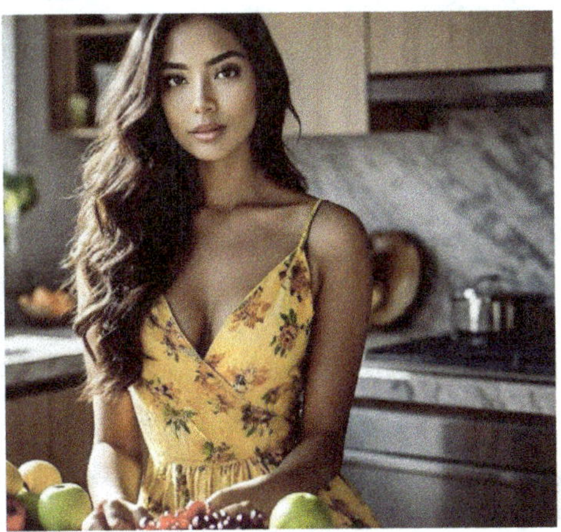

About The Book

In her new book, Endomorph Diet Plan For Men and Women Over 60, nutrition and wellness expert "Mary Williams" shares a comprehensive 90-day plan specifically tailored for mature adults looking to lose weight and improve their health as part of embracing vibrant aging.

As people enter their 60s and beyond, it becomes even more important to follow an anti-aging nutrition blueprint that supports the changing needs of the body. Yet standard diet plans often leave endomorph body types - who naturally carry more weight in the midsection - feeling discouraged and confused about the best strategies for their unique physiology.

In this book, Mary crafts a practical, sustainable plan that works with an endomorph's natural tendencies rather than against them. Readers will discover meal plans, recipes, shopping lists and lifestyle tips customized for their body type and stage of life. Mary's research-backed program focuses on balanced macronutrients, nutrient-dense whole foods and mindful eating to optimally support hormone levels, metabolism and overall wellness from within.

In addition to specific meal plans, the book includes 30 days of mindfulness exercises to bolster willpower and reduce stress eating. Mary also addresses common age-related health factors like mobility, medication use and chronic conditions to help custom-tailor the plan for each individual's needs. Filled with simple steps, this book provides everything busy aging adults need to lose weight, boost energy and take control of their health through embracing an endomorph-friendly lifestyle.

For men and women seeking a fresh approach to nutrition after 60, Mary Williams' Endomorph Diet Plan delivers practical strategies for addressing weight concerns and making vibrant aging a reality. Her realistic 90-day blueprint proves that you are never too old to improve wellness from the inside out.

Table Of Contents

Introduction

As an endomorph, diet and exercise should be approached with the understanding that what works for many people will not work for you.

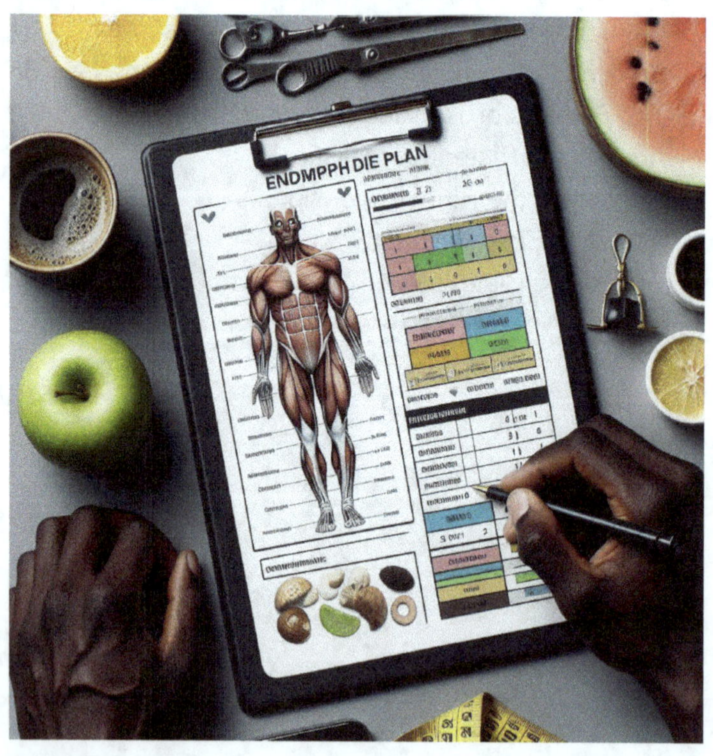

The recommendations that I am about to share about your endomorph diet plan and exercise strategy have the potential to make a significant impact on your endomorph weight loss efforts. However, it is important to understand that this is not a quick fix and adapting to the strategies I present here will take a strong commitment. This is also not a cookie-cutter approach, and I understand that there are varying degrees of endomorph body types. Some sources say endomorphs can also have mesomorph or ectomorph tendencies. Regardless of the shade of endomorph you are, if you identify yourself as an endomorph, this means your body possesses one of the three primary somatotypes. In this case, these strategies will be more effective for you compared to an ectomorph or mesomorph trying to lose weight.

When it comes to dieting and workout regimes, it is important for individuals to understand their metabolism and body type. This simple yet often overlooked component of weight loss is crucial in developing an effective plan to shed unwanted pounds and build muscle. This is especially the case when it comes to endomorph body types. In this recent publication, I shared how to determine if you are an endomorph body type and need some visual references.

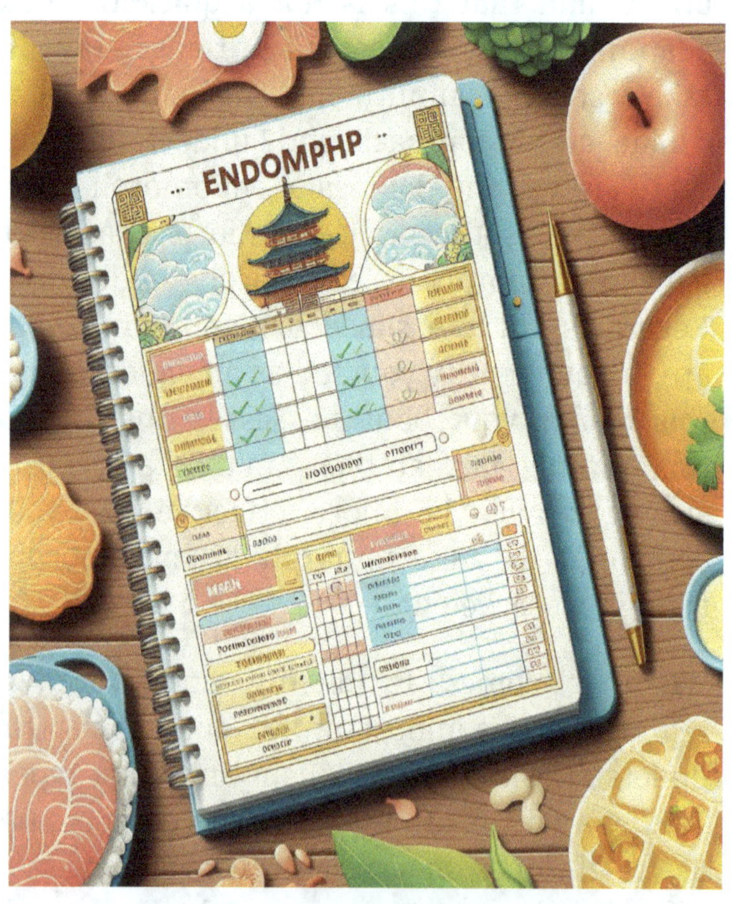

Understanding Endomorph Body Type

Only a small percentage of endomorphs will be able to stick with their diet and remain strict. There will be quite a few individuals that will fail to reach their goals. This may cause some to give up and revert back to old habits. It is important to avoid this from happening and just because results take longer for an endomorph to achieve, they will still be obtainable in the end. With enough dedication, discipline, and the right mindset, it is possible for an endomorph to transform their body by losing fat and being able to keep it off. Results will not be seen overnight but by making a change to lifestyle and sticking with a practical diet and training routine, an endomorph can achieve the healthier, more attractive body that they desire.

An endomorph is a male or female who is genetically predisposed to store fat easily and struggle to lose fat. This body type tends to be softer and rounder and has an appearance of being overweight. Due to a slower metabolism, it is difficult for endomorphs to lose weight. In order to lose fat, dieting will have to be strict, and most likely will have to be a lifestyle for the rest of their lives. An endomorph will have to pay more attention to the types of food they eat as well as the portion sizes. This is initially going to be hard for most as endomorphs typically will have poor eating habits. An effective diet for an endomorph is actually very similar to anyone else's diet. The only difference is that all diet plans will have to be more strict and less lenient. A typical diet will involve a macronutrient split of around 25% protein, 35% carbohydrate, and 30% fat. This can be adjusted slightly depending on the individual. All processed and junk food will have to be eliminated from the diet as well as any food high in saturated and trans fats. Endomorphs generally will have to eat more of their food earlier on in the day. This is because there is a higher chance that any food that is eaten later on in the day is more likely to be stored as fat. Eating carbs will help to stop an endomorph from craving foods that are not on a diet plan.

The more strict the diet plan is followed, the better the results will be. This may be hard at times because one may not get the results that they are looking for. This is to be expected of an endomorph.

With age comes various physiological changes in the body that can affect nutritional needs and ability to consume and digest certain foods. As people get older, their nutritional requirements tend to decrease compared to when they were younger. However, it's just as important for seniors to maintain good nutrition through a balanced diet in order to stay healthy and prevent age-related diseases and conditions. A tailored diet plan makes it easier for seniors to get the right nutrients and meet their dietary needs based on their individual health, lifestyle and any medical conditions they may have. This report will discuss in detail the key benefits of following a tailored diet plan for seniors.

Benefits of a tailored diet

1. Improved nutritional status

As people age, their nutritional needs change due to physiological changes taking place in the body. A tailored diet specifically designed for a senior's requirements can help them maintain optimal nutritional status. With a tailored plan, seniors can meet their daily requirements for calories, protein, vitamins, minerals and other essential nutrients. This helps prevent nutritional deficiencies that become more common with age. Some seniors may be at risk of not getting enough calories, protein or certain nutrients due to reduced appetite, chewing/swallowing difficulties, illnesses or social isolation. A personalized diet plan addresses these risks and ensures seniors get adequate nutrition.

2. Promotes healthy aging

Following a balanced diet tailored to their needs helps seniors stay healthy as they age. Good nutrition supports the normal functioning of all body systems and tissues. It promotes muscle strength, bone health, immune function, heart health, brain function and more. All of these factors directly influence healthy aging. A tailored diet plan provides seniors with the right combination and amounts of nutrients required to keep their bodies functioning optimally. This prevents accelerated aging effects and helps seniors actively engage in their daily lives even in their senior years. Good nutrition also lowers the risks of age-related chronic diseases and conditions like cardiovascular disease, type 2 diabetes, osteoporosis, arthritis etc.

3. Energy levels and physical functioning

A diet specifically formulated for a senior's needs can help boost their energy levels and overall physical functioning. As people get older, they tend to become less physically active due to reduced mobility, joint pains or other health issues. Good nutrition is important to supply the body with sufficient calories and high-quality protein to support daily activity and movement. A tailored diet provides seniors with enough energy to keep performing physical tasks and recreational activities independently without feeling tired or weak. Improved nutrition also promotes muscle strength, endurance and mobility - all of which impact a senior's quality of life and ability to function independently. This prevents accelerated physical and functional decline.

4. Supports disease management

Many seniors live with chronic health conditions like heart disease, diabetes, kidney disease etc. Following a tailored diet is beneficial for better disease management in such cases. Nutrition plans can be customized based on a senior's medical history, current medications, individual health goals and disease-specific dietary guidelines. For instance, a diet plan for diabetes would focus on careful carb and calorie control to manage blood sugar levels. Those with heart problems may require diets lower in sodium, saturated fat and cholesterol. Nutrition plans tailored to a senior's specific needs help control disease signs and symptoms, prevent complications and support treatment through therapeutic lifestyle changes and maintenance of a healthy weight. This not only promotes health but also reduces medical costs over the long term.

5. Supports medication use

Many seniors are dependent on daily medications to treat chronic conditions or simply as they age. Food and nutrients can impact how medications are absorbed and utilized in the body. A well-planned diet tailored to a senior's medication regime ensures there is no unwanted interaction between foods and drugs. It also prevents health issues arising due to taking medications on an empty stomach. For example, seniors on blood thinners like warfarin may need a diet consistent in vitamin K intake. Those with diabetes must coordinate medications and meals properly. A personalized nutrition plan for seniors guides appropriate meal timing and content for safe, effective medication use without side effects or health complications.

6. Supports independence

Good nutrition can play a role in maintaining independence for as long as possible among seniors. Nutritious, easily digestible food tailored to an individual's likes, dislikes and abilities support independent living. It avoids reliance on caregivers for assistance with eating. Well-planned meals and snacks help prevent fatigue, weakness and nutrition-related health issues that can potentially lead to loss of independence. For e.g. balanced, protein-rich soft foods support seniors with chewing/swallowing difficulties. Finger foods work for those with arthritis. Simple, pre-prepared meals suit seniors living alone. Appropriate diet adjustments empower seniors to look after their own needs and continue being self-sufficient for longer.

7. Supports brain health

Normal brain functioning is crucial for the emotional and social well-being of seniors. A tailored nutrition plan supports brain health and cognitive abilities through adequate intake of nutrients vital for neural health. These include antioxidants like vitamins C and E, B vitamins, omega-3 fatty acids, protein, iron, zinc and magnesium among others. Specific brain-healthy dietary patterns (e.g. Mediterranean diet) are also beneficial. Nutritious food helps prevent inflammation and cell damage linked to cognitive decline. Regular mental and social stimulation through activities combined with good nutrition have been shown to lower risks of dementia and Alzheimer's disease in older adults. This protects seniors from serious losses to their quality of life.

8. Improved mood and well-being

The gut-brain connection and effects of nutrition on neurochemistry are well documented. A diet tailored to meet nutritional needs of seniors supports positive mental wellness. Balanced, nutrient-rich meals regulate production of neurotransmitters like dopamine, serotonin and norepinephrine to lift mood. Adequate intake of omega-3s, B vitamins, magnesium, zinc and whole foods promote relaxation and calm. On the other hand, low blood sugar levels from missing/delaying meals can cause irritability. Fad diets or restrictive eating linked to certain nutrient deficiencies are also unhealthy for seniors' minds. A well-formulated nutrition plan providing balanced macros and micros keeps mood swings at bay and promotes overall psychological well-being among older adults.

9. Weight management

Both underweight and overweight impacts seniors' quality of life and health. A tailored diet aids in achieving and maintaining a healthy weight for better aging outcomes and disease prevention. Calorie goals appropriate for activity levels alongside nutrient-dense foods and limited excess prevent unwanted weight loss often seen in seniors due to declining appetite or lack of variety. For those who are overweight, a gradual weight loss plan protects lean muscle mass and promotes loss of excess body fat. This reduces burden on joints and the entire body. A personalized dietary approach reduces chronic disease risks and promotes independence, mobility and longevity for optimal senior living.

10. Managing appetite and diet preferences

Physiological changes and medication side effects often lower appetite among seniors. Boredom with repetitive foods can also affect nutritional intake negatively. A diet plan customized for a senior's personal tastes and preferences makes healthy eating more enjoyable and sustainable long-term. It incorporates favorite regional cuisines, favorite flavors from youth, cultural food rituals and comfort foods in moderation. Easy-to-eat low-effort options appeal to seniors more than difficult recipes. Nutritionally balanced mini-meals and snacks satisfy the appetite better than 3 large meals. Making suitable adjustments supports intake of necessary nutrients even in case of reduced appetite. This prevents undernutrition and associated health risks in seniors.

11. Cost-effective nutrition

Good nutrition need not always break the bank. A tailored diet plan for seniors guides cost-effective food choices based on budget, easy recipes, seasonal availability and pantry staples. Building meals around inexpensive protein sources like eggs, beans and lentils alongside in-season fruits-veggies provides balanced nutrition within budgets. Freeze-ahead homemade meals save money versus pre-cooked foods. Shopping discounted supermarket items rather than expensive specialty diets also helps. Planning grocery lists around weekly discounts prevents food waste. Nutritious home-cooked balanced fare proves significantly more cost-worth and accessible than expensive fad diets, processed convenience foods or frequent eating out. This promotes affordable healthy aging.

12. Social well-being

Sharing meals provides important social interactions and emotional fulfillment for many seniors. A tailored diet allows incorporating favorite traditional recipes of family/community in right proportions. Planning menus also supports seniors' participation in religious/cultural meal gatherings without compromising health. Well-balanced communal dishes appeal more than bland restricted options. Meal prepping and cooking together fosters bonds between seniors and caregivers. Diets accommodating dining partners' needs help seniors continue social meal traditions and maintain quality connections instead of feeling left out or dependent. Holistic wellness involves both physical and mental-social health benefits from good nutrition.

13. Supports oral health

Nutrition plays a role in oral hygiene which strongly impacts seniors' quality of life and dignity due to increased risk of dental problems and chewing difficulties. A tailored diet minimizes sticky/acidic foods that promote tooth decay and softens tough foods to aid chewing without strain. Nutritious smoothies are gentle on gums. Essentials like calcium and vitamin D from non-acidic sources support tooth/bone mineralization. Chewable nut butters/snacks deliver needed nourishment in easy-to-manage formats. Oral hygiene plans working with a dietitian support seniors in independent self-care for longer. This prevents serious dentition issues, infections and associated disabilities. Overall wellness involves both systemic and oral health considerations.

14. Prevent Malnutrition

As people age, their risk of malnutrition increases due to various factors like reduced appetite, chewing issues, financial constraints, isolation or illness. A tailored diet plan aims to meet all nutritional needs through smaller, frequent meals and nutrient-dense snacks. It focuses on high protein, calcium, vitamin D rich foods to prevent malnutrition-related disabilities. Compliance with the plan is tracked so corrective actions can be taken at the first signs of nutritional deficiencies developing. This helps seniors stay well-nourished and independent.

15. Supports Medical Conditions

Many seniors live with medical issues like diabetes, heart disease, kidney disease etc. Their diet needs to be planned carefully keeping these conditions in mind. A tailored meal plan considers medication schedules, individual health markers and disease-specific dietary advice. It ensures blood sugar/cholesterol levels, blood pressure, weight are managed well through therapeutic lifestyle changes. Following such a specialized nutrition routine supports seniors' medical treatment and overall well-being.

16. Improves GI Health

Slowed digestion is common in elderly , requiring softer, well-chewed foods in smaller portions. A tailored diet plan focuses on easily digestible high-fiber foods and fluids to support a healthy gastrointestinal system. It considers risks of constipation, diarrhea or acid reflux and guides management through appropriate menus. Maintaining GI health is important for seniors' comfort and nutritional status.

17. Enhances Dental Health

Good nutrition along with a dentist-approved dietary plan benefits senior dental hygiene. It focuses on non-sticky, non-acidic choices and chewier textures that don't strain teeth/jaws. Minerals like calcium protect fragile senior dentition from breakdown. Dietitian guidance prevents dental issues worsening other age-related conditions through proper nourishment.

18. Promotes Restful Sleep

Magnesium, calcium, vitamin D, healthy fats and carbohydrates in an optimized elder diet plan help relax the mind and body at bedtime. It identifies allergenic/stimulating foods to limit in evenings and makes sleep-friendly menu adjustments if any medications interfere with slumber. Maintaining quality sleep is crucial for senior wellness.

19. Fits Medical Budgets

A diet plan tailored to a senior's financial means focuses on affordable whole foods, discounted supermarket items, seasonal produce and home-cooked meals. It provides healthy balanced nutrition within medical/living budgets to support independent elder lifestyles through value-for-money suggestions.

Chapter 1: Assessing Your Health and Goals

Before diving headlong into a new nutrition plan, it is important to take stock of where you currently stand both physically and mentally. This chapter will guide you through an honest self-assessment of your weight, body composition, health markers and lifestyle habits. It also covers how to set appropriate goals for the next 90 days that motivate without setting unrealistic expectations. Let's start by taking a close look at your current health data points and priorities.

Evaluating Current Weight and Body Composition

The first step is obtaining an accurate read on your current weight status. Now while numbers on a scale alone do not define health, they do provide an objective baseline from which to measure progress. Make an appointment with your doctor for a full physical exam if it has been awhile. They can not only weigh you but assess factors like body mass index (BMI), waist circumference and body fat percentage for a complete picture:

- Use a digital scale at home daily to track fluctuations and average your weight over a week for your starting number.

- Note your height to calculate BMI via a chart. This indicates if you are underweight, normal, overweight or obese ranges.

- Measure your waist with a non-stretchable tape. A belly size over 35 inches for women or 40 inches for men signals increased disease risks.

- Ask your doctor about options like bioelectrical impedance analysis (BIA) or DEXA scans to precisely determine overall body fat percentage.

- Also take stock of factors like muscle tone, mobility, energy levels and how clothes are fitting currently.

While vanity metrics are not the goal, recording these baseline measurements provides data points to gauge 90-day improvements in body composition, not just scale weight. Regular tracking keeps you accountable while also identifying non-scale victories along the way.

Setting Realistic Weight Loss Goals

Now it's time to set practical short-term goals based on your starting health metrics. Losing too fast increases risks of nutritional deficiencies or regaining later. Aim for sustainable changes:

- Most health organizations recommend losing no more than 1-2 pounds per week for mature adults on a realistic calorie-controlled plan.

- Adjust goal weight loss down if you have significant health issues or limited mobility to prevent stress on your system.

- Also factor in body type tendencies like endomorphs losing more slowly than ectomorphs naturally.

- Set milestones like losing 5% of body weight as intermediate targets rather than focusing on pound numbers.

- Make lifestyle tweaks like increasing steps or water intake daily mini-goals as well to boost motivation.

- Remember weights fluctuate, so focus on directional trends rather than daily ups and downs.

- Be prepared to recalibrate goals if stalled to prevent frustration derailing your commitment.

With practical short-term targets in place, stay focused on health priorities over just vanity goals. Slower losses done sustainably lead to long-term changes.

Considering Health Conditions and Medications

Any existing medical issues require special attention, so review your diagnoses and treatments:

- Discuss your diet goals fully with your physician given conditions like diabetes, hypertension, digestive disorders etc.

- Ask how to complement and not contradict medications through lifestyle changes. For example, watch carb intake if using diabetes drugs.

- Note how certain drugs may impact weight like steroids, antidepressants and beta-blockers. Inform your doc of any bothersome side effects.

- Check for nutrient deficiencies if taking multiple prescriptions long-term as these can impact appetite and absorption.

- Be aware that combined chronic conditions multiply disease risks, so focus on recommended lifestyle therapies versus yo-yo dieting alone.

- Consider consulting a registered dietitian (RD) to help personalize your plan supporting any medical needs particularly.

Taking a multifaceted approach addressing underlying issues works much longer sustainably than quick fixes alone. With full transparency to your medical team, stay committed to regaining wellness from within safely.

Use this self-assessment phase to gain clarity on both your starting health baseline and motivations driving you towards embracing vibrant aging. While vanity has its place, focus above all on optimizing wellness holistically through realistic lifestyle changes. Maintain open communication with your healthcare providers, and feel empowered to customize your journey in a balanced, personalized way. You've got this! In the next chapter, we'll dive into the core nutritional foundations of the endomorph diet blueprint.

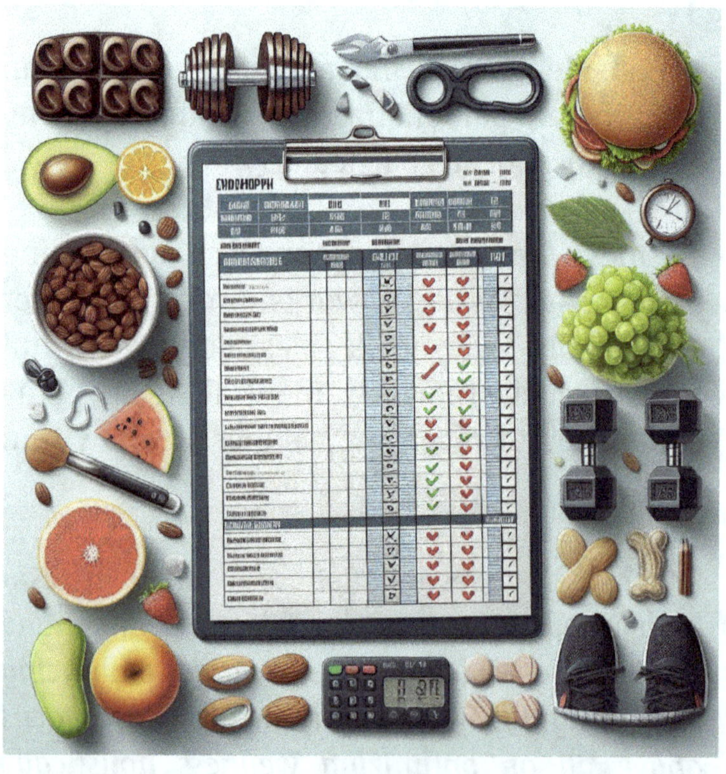

Chapter 2: Macronutrients and Micronutrients for Endomorphs

Now that we've assessed your current health and weight management priorities, let's dive into the core nutritional framework of this plan customized for your endomorph physiology. Understanding macronutrient and micronutrient needs for vibrant aging is essential to support both energy levels and metabolism long-term. In this chapter, we'll explore balancing carbohydrates, proteins and fats along with essential vitamins, minerals and hydration.

Balancing Carbohydrates, Proteins, and Fats

For endomorphs seeking to lose weight safely, finding the right macronutrient balance is key. Let's break this down:

- Carbohydrates: Aim for around 45-65% of daily calories from high-fiber, nutrient-dense complex carbs like fruits/veggies versus refined grains and sugars. These support stable blood sugar levels and metabolism.

- Proteins: Target 15-25% of calories from lean sources like chicken, fish, eggs, legumes and nuts/seeds. Proteins aid fullness and muscle mass critical as we age.

- Fats: Consume approximately 20-35% calories from healthy monounsaturated and polyunsaturated fats mainly. Limit saturated and trans fats which can promote increased abdominal weight gain over time.

- Adjust your intake based on your activity levels to maintain or lose weight at a reasonable 1-2 pounds per week as discussed in Chapter 2.

- Focus on balance as a lifestyle rather than being overly restrictive or harsh on yourself. Sustainability drives long-term success more than crash dieting or fasting.

Maintaining a balanced, fiber-rich calorie-controlled diet tailored to your metabolic needs will help promote gradual, long-lasting weight management and overall wellness.

Importance of Fiber and Hydration

Dietary fiber and hydration are worth special emphasis for endomorph health and mobility needs as we age:

- Fiber aids regularity which declines typically with age if not supplemented. It also promotes stable blood sugar levels and fullness to control overeating tendencies.

- Target a minimum of 25-30 grams of fiber daily from plant foods. Gradually work your way up to prevent intestinal discomfort as your system adjusts.

- Proper hydration also supports bodily functions like waste elimination along with lubricating joints for mobility.

- Drink half your body weight in ounces of water minimum daily (e.g. a 150 lb person drinks 75 ounces).

- In addition to water, enjoy herbal teas which provide beneficial plant compounds along with hydration and nutrients from homemade bone broths or fresh vegetable juices.

Maintaining regularity prevents constipation and its associated discomforts which commonly increase as we age. Fiber and water intake nourishes your system from within.

Incorporating Essential Vitamins and Minerals

A nutrient-dense whole foods diet along with a basic daily multivitamin/mineral supplement can help bridge any nutritional gaps in your diet for vibrant aging:

- Focus on antioxidant-rich fruits and vegetables which nourish cells and support immune function as free radical damage accumulates naturally as we age.

- Include lean proteins daily like eggs, fatty fish, nuts/seeds which provide satiating high-quality protein along with minerals like zinc, selenium and magnesium for metabolic and bone health.

- Healthy fats via olive oil, avocados, seeds, nuts and fatty fish supply fat-soluble vitamins A, D, E and K for hormonal balance and heart protection.

- Limit processed foods stripped of natural nutrients beneficial to the gastrointestinal tract microbiome which impacts mood and immunity.

Take a daily multivitamin/mineral supplement to supplement potential deficiencies from digestive changes, nutrient-depleting medications or other age-related issues. Choose whole foods as your primary source of nourishment however for optimal absorption.

Adhering to a balanced macronutrient and micronutrient-rich intake paired with proper hydration and fiber supports both weight management goals and overall vibrant health as we age. Use these nutritional foundations as a sustainable lifestyle focusing on permanent wellness improvements from the inside out. In the next chapter, we'll dive into specific meal planning strategies and recipes tailored for endomorph metabolism.

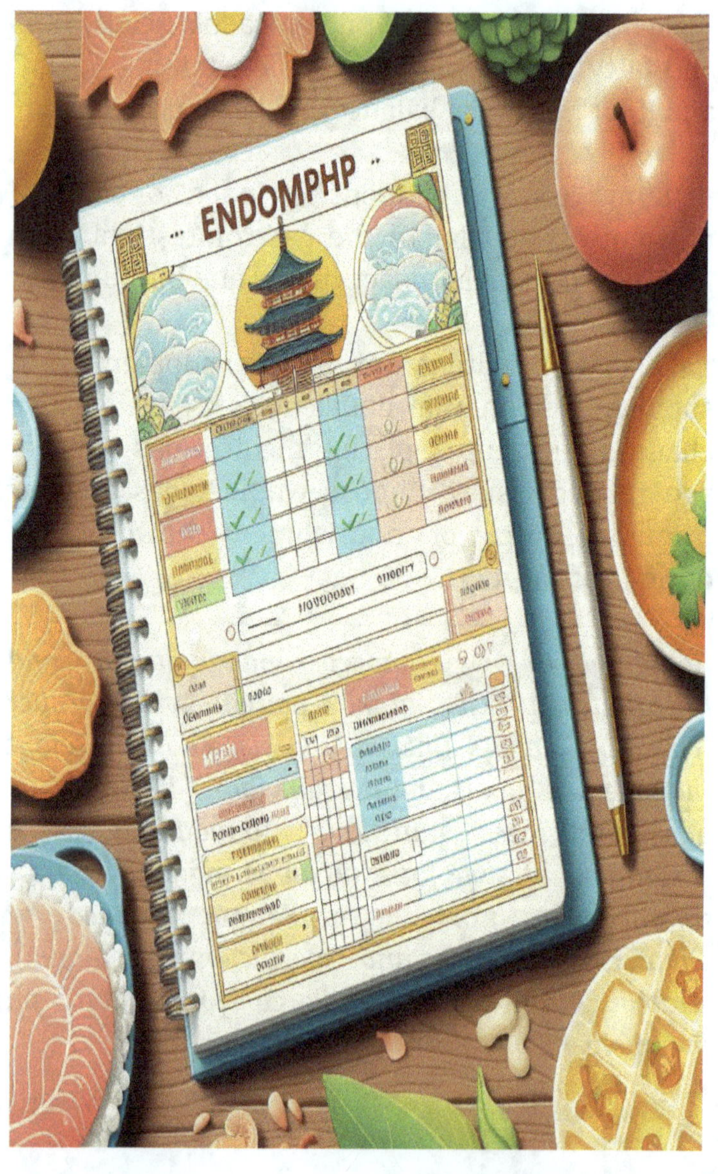

Chapter 3: Meal Planning and Portion Control

Now that we've reviewed the core macronutrient and micronutrient requirements for vibrant aging as an endomorph, it's time to apply this framework through practical and sustainable meal planning. This chapter focuses on balancing meals intelligently, controlling servings for weight loss support and selecting snacks to maintain steadiness between meals. Let's begin strategizing our nutrition!

Creating a Balanced Meal Plan

Developing weekly menus ensures a variety of satisfying whole foods without overwhelm or uncertainty:

- Incorporate at least 3-4 fruits/veggies, 2-3 lean proteins and healthy fats per meal for balanced macros and micros.

- Focus one-third of plates on starch/grain sources ideally at each sitting for balanced energy release.

- Prepare double batches on weekends like soups/stews for easy meal prep going forward.

- Consider mix-and-match meal pairings and leftovers throughout the week for convenience.

- Do not skip meals which can disrupt your metabolism and lead to overindulging later.

- Stay flexible and make sustainable adjustments as needed based on your schedule.

Meal mapping takes the guesswork out of nutrition while supplying your unique needs daily for fast, balanced weight management success.

Controlling Portion Sizes for Weight Management

For the endomorph physiology seeking to lose weight long-term, controlling portions through mindful techniques is key:

- Weigh and measure food amounts initially until you have a grasp of standard serving estimations for Macs, proteins and fats.

- Use smaller plates to make moderate servings appear abundant which satiates more than skimpy amounts.

- Fill half plates with low-cal veggie options instead of topping them off with grains/starches for bigger meals while sticking to calorie limits.

- Focus on fiber/protein/fat rich whole foods, and limit liquid calories frequently overlooked but harder to regulate intake of.

- Factor in occasional balanced snacks/treats discussed in section 3 while keeping meals mindfully portioned.

With patient practice, mindful portion control paired with a balanced meal plan sustains metabolism while addressing overconsumption tendencies for lasting results.

Snack Ideas for Sustained Energy

In addition to your major meals, snacking keeps blood sugar and energy steady without ruining your calorie balance for the day:

- Choose nutrient-dense portable snacks like nuts, seeds, nut butters with fruits or veggies, hard boiled eggs, Greek yogurt or cheese and crackers.

- Avoid calorie-dense empty carb options like pastries, chips, candy etc. which disrupt blood sugar levels and promote excess hunger/cravings later.

- If dining out, look for filling protein-centric appetizers, salads/soups over comfort carbs/desserts to stay feeling sated.

- Stay hydrated with herbal tea or water between meals to distinguish true hunger signals from thirst often misinterpreted.

Balanced snacking provides nutrition that supports your weight management goals when mindfully timed and portioned into your daily calorie count.

Developing a regular whole foods-based meal plan, controlling reasonable portions through mindful tools and focusing on balanced low glycemic snacking supplies your body continuously without sabotaging your efforts. Consistency sustains your momentum while flexibility keeps you on track permanently. Let's now dive into applying these strategies through practical and delicious endomorph-friendly recipes.

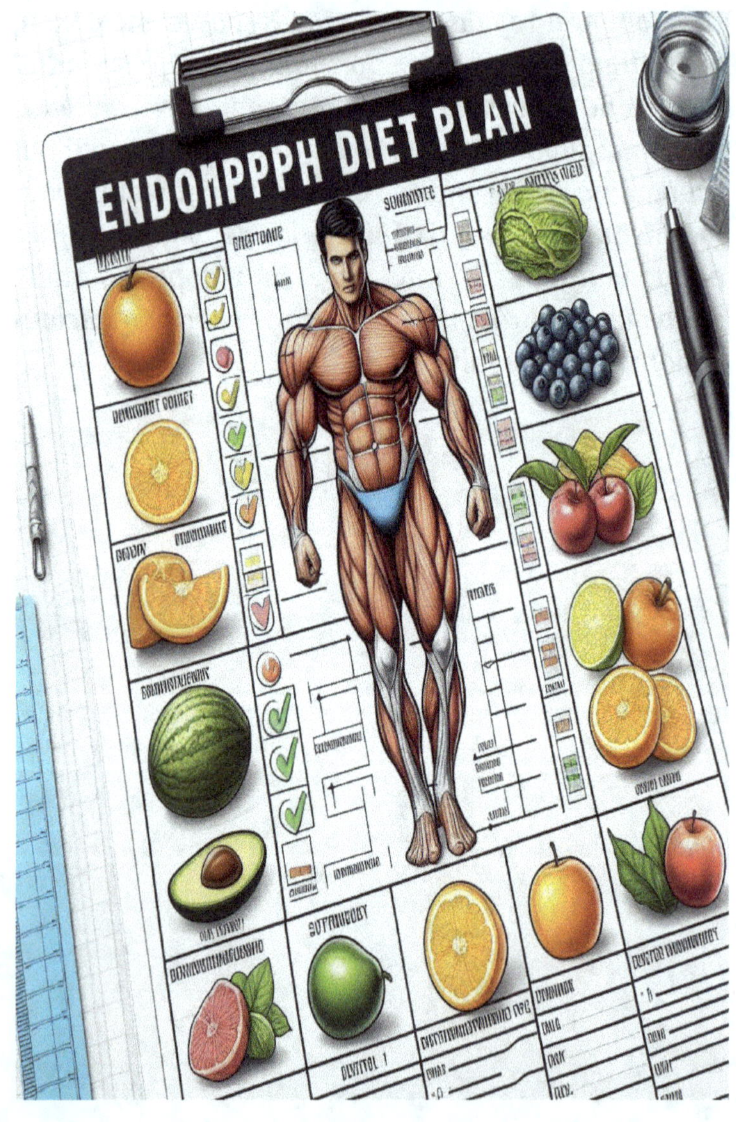
ENDOMPPPH DIET PLAN

Chapter 5: Strategies for Weight Loss and Metabolism Boost

While nutrition serves as the foundation for health, complimenting your meal plan with physical activity strategies can boost your weight management results even further. This chapter explores incorporating safe and effective exercise routines tailored for the endomorph body type seeking metabolism and energy level improvements.

Incorporating Regular Physical Activity

Research clearly shows exercise supports weight loss for mature adults when combined with calorie control:

- Aim for a minimum of 150 minutes of moderate activity like brisk walking or water exercise per week per guidelines.

- Break it up into 30 minutes a day, 5 days a week for balanced and sustainable fitness habits long-term.

- Do what feels enjoyable for you like gardening, dancing, yoga or strength training using light weights 2-3 times weekly additionally.

- Start low and go slow to prevent injury as movement needs typically decline with age gradually if not addressed.

- Focus on exercises your body can safely handle versus potentially risky high-impact options. Check with your doctor as needed.

Regular movement nourishes your muscles, bones, mind and metabolism when effort is made gradually enjoyable versus punishing routines unsustainable long-term.

High-Intensity Interval Training for Endomorphs

Short bursts of conditioning intervals provide metabolism boosting benefits when incorporated gently 1-2 times weekly for endomorphs:

- Perform intervals indoors if weather prohibits like marching in place, jogging on a treadmill or spinning stationary bike.

- Start with 30 seconds of moderate effort followed by 90 seconds of lighter recovery up to 10 cycles over 20-30 minutes 2 times weekly.

- Modify intervals to a comfortable challenge level based on your fitness and mobility limitations safely with guidance from certified professionals as needed.

- Replenish glycogen stores with a balanced recovery snack containing carbs and proteins afterwards.

Done judiciously, interval training supplies metabolic benefits without joint/impact risks when paced properly for continued long-term weight management adherence.

Tips for Increasing Metabolic Rate

Additional lifestyle adjustments support your body's innate calorie and fat burning potential:

- Prioritize quality sleep nightly which impacts hunger hormone balance regulating appetite and weight.

- Manage stress through mindfulness methods like yoga, deep breathing, relaxation techniques shown to lower cortisol levels driving belly fat storage.

- Expose yourself to natural light/vitamin D daily which influences hundreds of genes related to metabolism, immunity and mood.

- Drink water throughout the day versus caloric beverages keeping your system hydrated for optimal digestive function.

- Exercising with a friend increases motivation and commitment versus solo sessions easily skipped.

Maximizing your metabolism works synergistically with a balanced lifestyle preventing plateaus for continued fat loss and wellness benefits.

Incorporating sustainable physical activity through enjoyable exercises tailored to your abilities supplements your nutrition efforts for amplified weight management results. Use movement to nourish both your muscles and mood while taking a holistic approach addressing innate metabolic drivers. Consistency with changes over time cultivates enduring health improvements and quality of life as an endomorph aging vibrantly. On to applying it all!

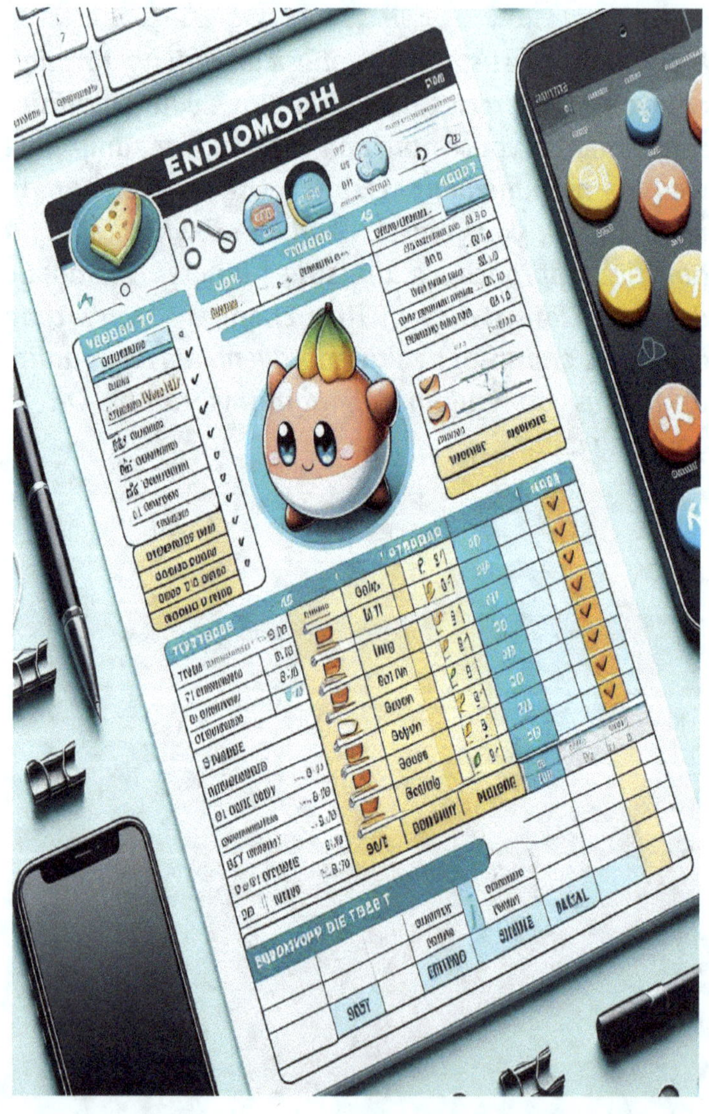

Chapter 6: Managing Hunger and Cravings

While your diet plan supplies balanced nourishment, learning hunger versus craving signals eases navigating mindless eating tendencies often challenging for endomorphs. This chapter explores mindful approaches distinguishing physical hunger from emotional triggers. Understanding your needs supports sustainable changes without strict deprivation.

Understanding Hunger Signals

Distinguishing true physiological hunger from habitual snacking requires patience:

- Pay attention to early hunger pangs versus waiting until ravenous to refuel which primes overeating habits harder to regulate.

- Drink a full glass of water first which often masks mild hunger effectively while hydrating and filling space in the stomach mildly.

- Note when hunger appears versus when stress/boredom sets in prompting food habits passed for nourishment.

- If not truly hungry within 30 minutes, try distracting yourself with other healthy coping mechanisms until the next scheduled small meal or snack time.

With self-awareness, you can nip unnecessary eating triggers in the bud before rationalizing overconsumption to yourself non-nutritive needs.

Healthy Snack Options to Curb Cravings

Mindful snacking between balanced meals prevents cravings from snowballing:

- Prepare crunchy veggies with hummus or nut butter for dipping, cut up fruits, a hardboiled egg or piece of cheese with whole grain crackers to satisfy light hunger satiating yet calorically moderately.

- Roasted chickpeas or other beans make a tasty high-fiber snack as well controlling blood sugar when paired with a lean protein.

- Homemade popsicles using fruit purees supply hydration and nutrients cooling down without excess sugar of store-bought versions.

With nutritious options on hand as needed, you can redirect oral fixation tendencies onto wholesome foods satisfying actual nourishment requirements versus emotional reliance on indulgences.

Mindful Eating Techniques

Developing awareness around consuming food intentionally supports dietary success:

- Practice sitting down to eat without distractions allowing yourself to focus completely on flavors and fullness signals.

- Chew food mindfully until it is liquidized fully in your mouth aiding proper digestion while fostering appreciation for your nourishment.

- Stop eating the moment you feel fullness discomfort versus cleaning your plate out of routine, potentially overriding internal cues.

- Pay attention to how different foods make you feel energy level and digestion wise helping identify agreeable options.

- Do not deny yourself enjoyable treats either but thoughtfully factor limited indulgences into your overall well-portioned calorie balance.

With discipline and routine, mindful eating habits become second nature improving your relationship with food permanently. In the next chapter, let's discuss addressing emotional eating triggers holistically.

Here is a continued draft of Chapter 6 professionally explaining additional mindfulness techniques:

While understanding physical hunger and craving triggers aids managing eating behaviors, integrating mindfulness more holistically supports lifestyle changes seamlessly. Let's explore complementary mind-body practices.

Developing Self-Awareness through Mindfulness

Conquering emotional reliance on food requires self-reflection to discern root causes. Mindfulness cultivates present-moment awareness diminishing reactivity:

- Daily journaling prompts identifying situational emotions, automatic thoughts and alternative coping actions modeled.

- Guided meditation utilizing breathing and body scans taught relaxing the mind from ruminations fueling overeating urges.

- Affirmation writing exercise reprogramming subconscious biases like "I always feel out of control around sweets' ' reframed positively.

- Progressive muscle relaxation and imagery scripts provided tensing then relaxing each muscle group whilst visualizing stress leave the body.

Pairing Inner Wisdom with Outer Support

A compassionate, non-judgmental inner dialogue nourishes behavior shifts versus harsh self-talk maintaining patterns. Community also motivates:

- Accountability partnerships establish check-ins keeping practitioners responsible to goals sensitively.

- Online forums connecting individuals build rapport relieving isolation exacerbating emotional eating tendencies.

- Professional counseling may benefit some unpacking underlying factors behind compulsive habits resolved effectively.

Adopting mindfulness cultivates self-knowledge guiding intuitive nourishment aligned with one's highest well-being. While willpower influences behaviors initially, integrating mindfulness transforms self-sabotage at root levels permanently. With continued practice and community, one learns flexibility adapting to life's ever-changing circumstances harmoniously.

Mindfulness in Daily Life

Integrating brief mindfulness practices into everyday routines supports addressing triggers as they arise:

- Deep breathing exercises practiced before and after meals dissipate stress hormones impairing appetite regulation.

- Short walking or mind-body meditation breaks replenish energy stores drained from overwhelm promoting unhealthy escapism.

- Compassionate self-talk and affirmations restructured reframing negative thought distortions fueling emotional distress.

- Gratitude journaling highlighted three things appreciated each day shifting focus from lack externally or internally.

- Pleasant sensory awareness of nature engaged the five senses reconnecting to inner calm replacing distractions numbing emotions.

\- Yoga or stretching sequences incorporate mindfulness of bodily sensations lessening discomfort perpetuating overindulgence habits.

Addressing triggers in real-time rather than retrospection alone.

The Ripple Effect of Mindfulness

Mindfulness diffuses distress across one's entire existence by cultivating acceptance:

\- Self-care expanded beyond dieting to nurturing all life domains nourishing overall well-being eliminating discontented eating fixations.

\- Interpersonal relationships benefited from improved empathy, communication and emotional regulation repairing social ties and strengthening coping strategies.

\- Career or family responsibilities managed efficiently with clarity rather than stress-fueled scarcity mindsets alleviating triggers of consuming compulsively.

\- Environmental contributions engaged giving back out of compassion for all life enhancing self-worth beyond weight or appearance enhancing longevity.

By addressing the whole self, one liberates from dependencies and embraces balance seamlessly responding skillfully to whatever arises.

By understanding your authentic physical needs versus learned behavioral habits, you empower yourself to make sustainable nourishment choices addressing hunger satisfaction versus craving escapism. Developing mindfulness around eating aids long-term lifestyle success adaptable to any stage of life more holistically. Let's now explore nourishment of your whole being further.

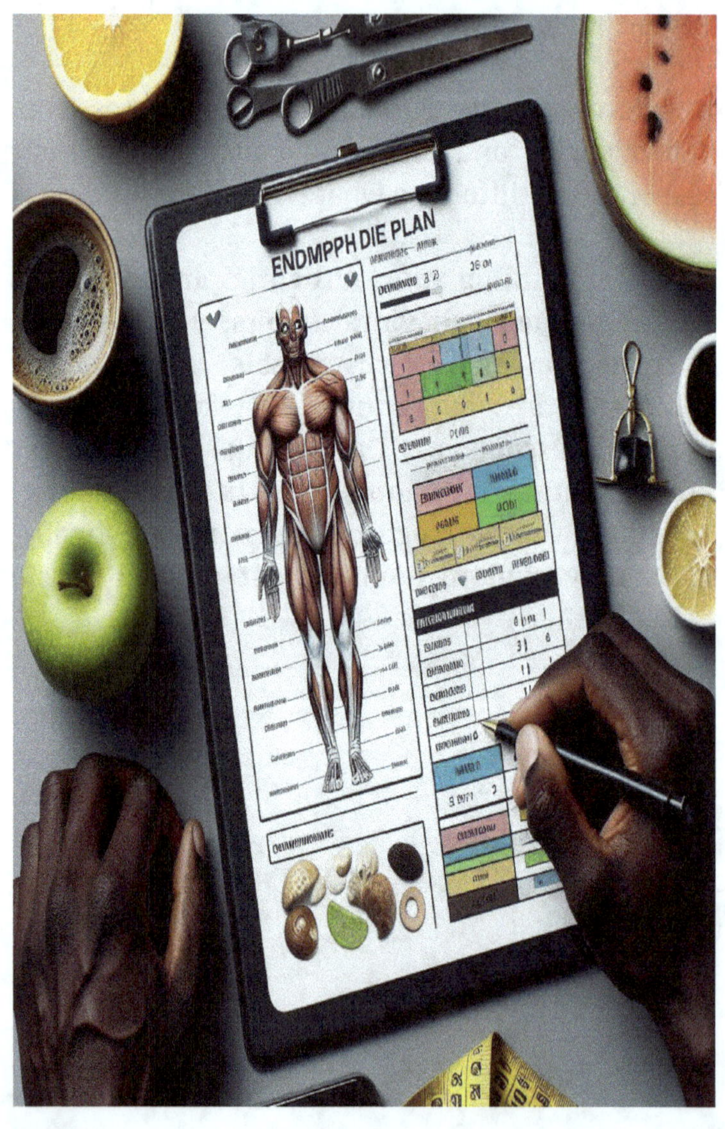

Chapter 8: Tracking Progress and Adjusting the Plan

While consistency fuels results, monitoring your efforts objectively aids maintaining motivation through obstacles inevitable in any health journey. This chapter discusses tools for evaluating physiological changes and recognizing stalling effectively. Continuous improvement cultivates long-term success.

Monitoring Weight and Body Measurements

Periodic self-assessments gauge effectiveness without fixation on daily fluctuations:

- Weigh yourself 1-2 times weekly at most ideally on waking before eating/drinking using the same scale for accuracy.

- Jot pounds lost, fat lost, muscle gained or other metrics determined by your doctor or fitness tracker reliably.

- Also note waist, hip and bust measurements monthly ideally using a non-stretchable tape to assess body composition shifts specifically.

- Photos capture subtle changes and mirrors may miss reassuring you of non-scale accomplishments like increased strength/mobility.

- Track NSVs (non-scale victories) beside numbers appreciating holistic benefits beyond just the numbers on the scale.

Objective yet flexible evaluation encourages without obsessiveness setting you up for sustainable lifestyle maintenance.

Recognizing Plateaus and Making Adjustments

Stalling signals requiring tweaks periodically:

- If weight loss slows to less than 0.5 lbs weekly for a month despite adherence, adjust calorie intake down slightly by 100-200 calories.

- Plateaus often occur naturally after significant losses from water weight so maintain patience and consistency for 4-6 weeks typically before significant changes.

- Consider logging food and activities daily for a week pinpointing portions creeping up or exercises slacking to reassume accountability.

- If health issues have changed, consult your doctor regarding potential medication adjustments to impact metabolism.

- Incorporate an additional weekly high-intensity interval training session or short walk after meals raising baseline metabolism gently.

With small targeted remedies, you can push past hiccups resuming momentum accomplished gradually without crisis or deprivation.

Seeking Professional Guidance when Needed

**While this guide provides a solid foundation, certain scenarios require expert input:**

- Consult your physician if weight loss stalls completely for 3+ months despite adjustments; underlying factors may need evaluation.

- Meet with a Registered Dietitian if you are struggling with cravings, hunger or disordered thinking patterns jeopardizing your welfare psychologically or physically.

- Consider nutritional counseling if managing multiple chronic diseases, disabilities or special dietary needs beyond a self-directed program.

- Seek medical clearance before beginning an intense exercise program if you have uncontrolled medical issues, injuries or mobility limitations precariously.

Appropriate expert support preserves health optimizing results professionally when ambiguity arises outside of your experience level.

The Benefits of Tracking for Awareness

Rather than strict self-evaluation, recording intake/progress builds self-knowledge optimizing efforts long-term:

- Nutritional logging identifies portion sizes creeping up or macronutrient imbalances adjusted restoring momentum.

- Activity tracking monitors exercise/movement habits slacking without full realization disrupted.

- Metrics provide perspective recognizing natural plateaus rather than immutable failure with continuous learning empowering adaptability.

- Journaling expressions/emotions around food associates situational cues prompting mindless habits changed constructively.

- Patterns inform personalized modifications catered to one's unique biology maximizing results supportively.

Addressing Plateaus Realistically

Minor tweaks revive results avoiding drastic measures counterproductive:

- Adding 10 minutes daily activity multiplies benefits slightly revving metabolism modestly.

- Exchanging higher calorie ingredients tweaks 100-200 intake calms cravings gently.

- Stress management tools alleviate cortisol driving urges without overhauling responsibilities or social commitments.

- Adequate hydration and nutrition optimize performance supportively versus dehydration fatiguing discipline.

Focusing on Wellness, Not Just Weight

Benefits expand beyond vanity nourishing whole-self confidence long-term:

- Exercise boosts mood, sleep, mobility and immune function significantly influencing longevity holistically.

- Nutritious eating supports disease prevention, mental clarity and energy levels impacting quality of living dramatically.

- Self-care reduces injury risks, complications and medical costs from inactivity, stress or unhealthy dependencies protecting well-being fiscally.

- Healthier patrons motivate spouses, children, coworkers and communities uplifting public health exponentially.

Consulting the Right Professionals

<u>Specific issues warrant specialized guidance:</u>
- Dietitians assess micronutrient levels, disordered eating thoughts or special dietary requirements like diabetes individualizing support.

- Physical therapists treat injuries possibly hindering safe exercise progression or identify alternative range-of-motion options.

- Nurse practitioners screen for undiagnosed conditions influencing metabolism managed optimally.

- Psychologists help parse emotional eating triggers, set healthy expectations or cope with underlying stressors holistically.

Adjusting Expectations Gradually

True maintenance means ongoing nourishment, not deprivation:

- Steady improvements inspire as progress naturally decelerates, not stalls, with long-term commitment to balanced self-care.

- Small losses still signify fat replacement with muscle or enhanced body composition seen in mirrors, not numbers alone.

- Non-scale benefits prove motivation outweighing vanity like increased mobility, confidence or disease prevention significantly.

Embracing Plateaus and Ups/Downs

<u>Flexibility prevents burnout sticking with healthy routines:</u>

- Weekly highs and lows average out over time viewed less strictly than daily water weight fluctuations.

- Being kind yet accountable preserves motivation hitting occasional bumps, not used as excuses.

- Celebrating non-scale achievements nourishes well-being beyond just aesthetics through plateaus uplifting.

By tracking purposefully yet uncritically, one cultivates resilience navigating inevitable curves gracefully healthfully for life. Continuous small refinements enact enormous positive change.

Your health journey is a lifelong process of continual learning and improvement, not a short-term destination. Approaching progress supportively through awareness instead of judgment cultivates resilience and self-compassion.

While dedication brings results, flexibility mitigates burnout recognizing life's ebbs and flows. Small but consistent optimizations compound significantly over time, far surpassing radical restriction's sustainability.

Seeking wisdom from reliable sources like medical experts ensures issues receive proper attention. But ultimately your care is self-directed - trust your inner guidance and don't hesitate to tailor plans meeting your changing needs.

Wellness encompasses vibrant aging of the whole self beyond just physical metrics. Nourishing community, purpose, self-care and relationships as diligently as activities/nutrition celebrates life fully.

Challenges will come. Yet through patience, adaptability and celebrating non-scale wins, motivation perseveres inspiring continual learning and improvement - the truest marks of an optimized lifestyle seamlessly navigating life's curves.

With supportively guided effort and compassion for the journey, not just outcomes, sustained healthy habits blossom naturally as your unique and worthy self shines through. Your greatest gift lies ahead in receiving each phase of life gratefully. Onward to vibrant living!

Maintaining accountability fuels lasting progress. Learn from plateaus and use feedback constructively avoiding all-or-nothing thinking. With patience and adjustments as needed, you cultivate resilience handling curves gracefully along your vibrant aging journey. Continued small successes build enormous fulfillment and well-being lifetimes. Let's move forward confidently!

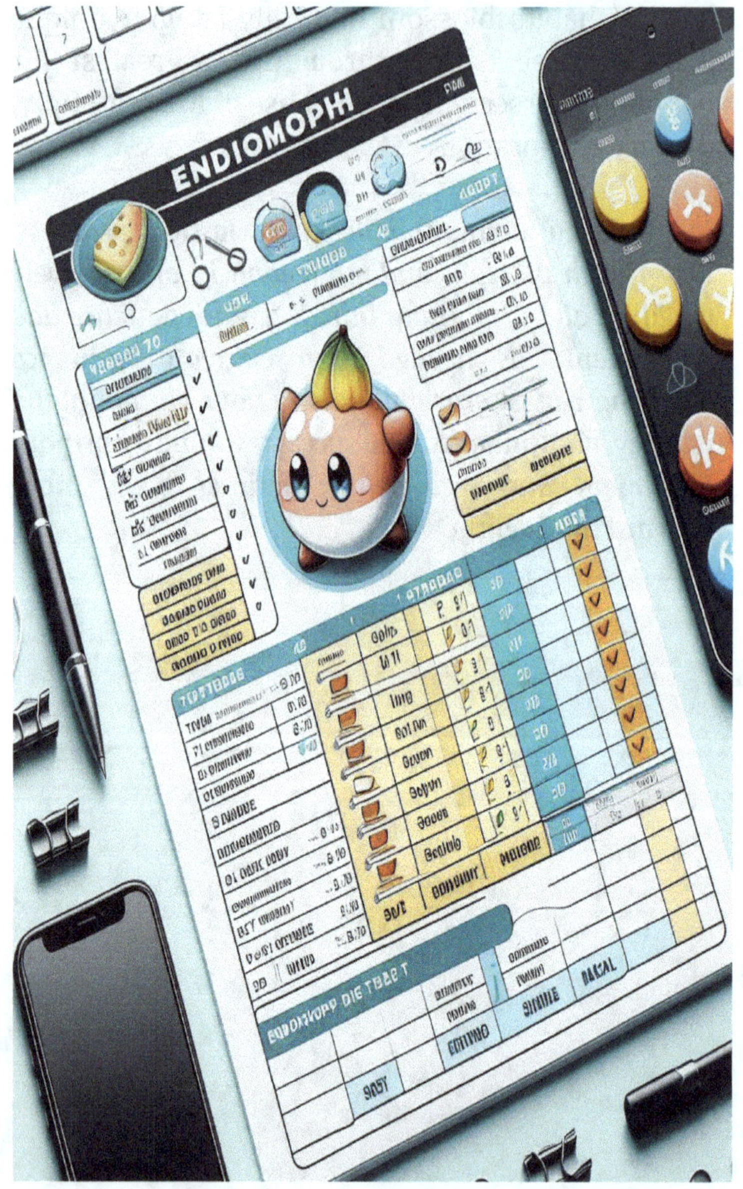

Exclusive Tracking tools

My fitness Goals Tracker

MY FITNESS GOALS TRACKER

Starting Date: Ending Date:

My Top Fitness Goals

Motivation:

Bad Habits to Cut

Start   Goal

Good Habits to Keep

Chest

Arm

Waist

Hips

BMI

Weight

Body Fat

Muscle

MY FITNESS GOALS TRACKER

Starting Date:

Ending Date:

My Top Fitness Goals

Motivation:

Start	Goal	
		Chest
		Arm
		Waist
		Hips
		BMI
		Weight
		Body Fat
		Muscle

Bad Habits to Cut

Good Habits to Keep

MY FITNESS GOALS TRACKER

Starting Date: **Ending Date:**

My Top Fitness Goals

Motivation:

Start	Goal	
		Chest
		Arm
		Waist
		Hips
		BMI
		Weight
		Body Fat
		Muscle

Bad Habits to Cut

Good Habits to Keep

MY FITNESS GOALS TRACKER

Starting Date: **Ending Date:**

My Top Fitness Goals

Motivation:

Bad Habits to Cut

Good Habits to Keep

Start   **Goal**

Chest

Arm

Waist

Hips

BMI

Weight

Body Fat

Muscle

MY FITNESS GOALS TRACKER

Starting Date: **Ending Date:**

My Top Fitness Goals

Motivation:

Start   **Goal**

Bad Habits to Cut

| Chest |
| Arm |
| Waist |
| Hips |
| BMI |
| Weight |
| Body Fat |
| Muscle |

Good Habits to Keep

MY FITNESS GOALS TRACKER

Starting Date:

Ending Date:

My Top Fitness Goals

Bad Habits to Cut

Good Habits to Keep

Motivation:

Start	Goal	
		Chest
		Arm
		Waist
		Hips
		BMI
		Weight
		Body Fat
		Muscle

MY FITNESS GOALS TRACKER

Starting Date:

Ending Date:

My Top Fitness Goals

Motivation:

Start   **Goal**

Chest

Arm

Waist

Hips

BMI

Weight

Body Fat

Muscle

Bad Habits to Cut

Good Habits to Keep

MY FITNESS GOALS TRACKER

Starting Date:

Ending Date:

My Top Fitness Goals

Motivation:

Start **Goal**

Bad Habits to Cut

Good Habits to Keep

Chest

Arm

Waist

Hips

BMI

Weight

Body Fat

Muscle

MY FITNESS GOALS TRACKER

Starting Date:

Ending Date:

My Top Fitness Goals

Motivation:

Start

Goal

Bad Habits to Cut

Good Habits to Keep

- Chest
- Arm
- Waist
- Hips
- BMI
- Weight
- Body Fat
- Muscle

MY FITNESS GOALS TRACKER

Starting Date:

Ending Date:

My Top Fitness Goals

Motivation:

Start

Goal

Bad Habits to Cut

Good Habits to Keep

- Chest
- Arm
- Waist
- Hips
- BMI
- Weight
- Body Fat
- Muscle

MY FITNESS GOALS TRACKER

Starting Date: **Ending Date:**

My Top Fitness Goals

Motivation:

Start	Goal

Bad Habits to Cut

Good Habits to Keep

- Chest
- Arm
- Waist
- Hips
- BMI
- Weight
- Body Fat
- Muscle

MY FITNESS GOALS TRACKER

Starting Date:

Ending Date:

My Top Fitness Goals

Motivation:

Start	Goal

Bad Habits to Cut

Good Habits to Keep

Chest

Arm

Waist

Hips

BMI

Weight

Body Fat

Muscle

MY FITNESS GOALS TRACKER

Starting Date: **Ending Date:**

My Top Fitness Goals

Motivation:

Start	Goal

Bad Habits to Cut

Good Habits to Keep

Chest

Arm

Waist

Hips

BMI

Weight

Body Fat

Muscle

MY FITNESS GOALS TRACKER

Starting Date:

Ending Date:

My Top Fitness Goals

Motivation:

Start	Goal	
		Chest
		Arm
		Waist
		Hips
		BMI
		Weight
		Body Fat
		Muscle

Bad Habits to Cut

Good Habits to Keep

MY FITNESS GOALS TRACKER

Starting Date:

Ending Date:

My Top Fitness Goals

Motivation:

Start   **Goal**

Bad Habits to Cut

Good Habits to Keep

Chest

Arm

Waist

Hips

BMI

Weight

Body Fat

Muscle

My Fitness Challenge Tracker

FITNESS CHALLENGE

Month: **Week of:**

	Exercise/Workout	Sets & Reps
S		
M		
T		
W		
T		
F		
S		

Notes:

FITNESS CHALLENGE

Month: **Week of:**

	Exercise/Workout	Sets & Reps
S		
M		
T		
W		
T		
F		
S		

Notes:

FITNESS CHALLENGE

Month: **Week of:**

	Exercise/Workout	Sets & Reps
S		
M		
T		
W		
T		
F		
S		

Notes:

FITNESS CHALLENGE

Month: **Week of:**

	Exercise/Workout	Sets & Reps
S		
M		
T		
W		
T		
F		
S		

Notes:

FITNESS CHALLENGE

Month: **Week of:**

	Exercise/Workout	Sets & Reps
S		
M		
T		
W		
T		
F		
S		

Notes:

FITNESS CHALLENGE

Month: **Week of:**

	Exercise/Workout	Sets & Reps
S		
M		
T		
W		
T		
F		
S		

Notes:

FITNESS CHALLENGE

Month: **Week of:**

	Exercise/Workout	Sets & Reps
S		
M		
T		
W		
T		
F		
S		

Notes:

FITNESS CHALLENGE

Month: **Week of:**

	Exercise/Workout	Sets & Reps
S		
M		
T		
W		
T		
F		
S		

Notes:

FITNESS CHALLENGE

Month: **Week of:**

	Exercise/Workout	Sets & Reps
S		
M		
T		
W		
T		
F		
S		

Notes:

FITNESS CHALLENGE

Month: **Week of:**

	Exercise/Workout	Sets & Reps
S		
M		
T		
W		
T		
F		
S		

Notes:

FITNESS CHALLENGE

Month: **Week of:**

	Exercise/Workout	Sets & Reps
S		
M		
T		
W		
T		
F		
S		

Notes:

FITNESS CHALLENGE

Month: **Week of:**

	Exercise/Workout	Sets & Reps
S		
M		
T		
W		
T		
F		
S		

Notes:

FITNESS CHALLENGE

Month: **Week of:**

	Exercise/Workout	Sets & Reps
S		
M		
T		
W		
T		
F		
S		

Notes:

FITNESS CHALLENGE

Month: **Week of:**

	Exercise/Workout	Sets & Reps
S		
M		
T		
W		
T		
F		
S		

Notes:

FITNESS CHALLENGE

Month: **Week of:**

	Exercise/Workout	Sets & Reps
S		
M		
T		
W		
T		
F		
S		

Notes:

My Calories Tracker

CALORIES TRACKER

Month: **Week of:**

	Breakfast	Lunch	Dinner	Snack
Sun				
Mon				
Tue				
Wed				
Thu				
Fri				
Sat				

CALORIES TRACKER

Month: **Week of:**

	Breakfast	Lunch	Dinner	Snack
Sun				
Mon				
Tue				
Wed				
Thu				
Fri				
Sat				

CALORIES TRACKER

Month: **Week of:**

	Breakfast	Lunch	Dinner	Snack
Sun				
Mon				
Tue				
Wed				
Thu				
Fri				
Sat				

CALORIES TRACKER

Month: **Week of:**

	Breakfast	Lunch	Dinner	Snack
Sun				
Mon				
Tue				
Wed				
Thu				
Fri				
Sat				

CALORIES TRACKER

Month: **Week of:**

	Breakfast	Lunch	Dinner	Snack
Sun				
Mon				
Tue				
Wed				
Thu				
Fri				
Sat				

CALORIES TRACKER

Month: Week of:

	Breakfast	Lunch	Dinner	Snack
Sun				
Mon				
Tue				
Wed				
Thu				
Fri				
Sat				

CALORIES TRACKER

Month: **Week of:**

	Breakfast	Lunch	Dinner	Snack
Sun				
Mon				
Tue				
Wed				
Thu				
Fri				
Sat				

CALORIES TRACKER

Month: **Week of:**

	Breakfast	Lunch	Dinner	Snack
Sun				
Mon				
Tue				
Wed				
Thu				
Fri				
Sat				

CALORIES TRACKER

Month: Week of:

	Breakfast	Lunch	Dinner	Snack
Sun				
Mon				
Tue				
Wed				
Thu				
Fri				
Sat				

CALORIES TRACKER

Month: **Week of:**

	Breakfast	Lunch	Dinner	Snack
Sun				
Mon				
Tue				
Wed				
Thu				
Fri				
Sat				

CALORIES TRACKER

Month: ____________________   Week of: ____________________

	Breakfast	Lunch	Dinner	Snack
Sun				
Mon				
Tue				
Wed				
Thu				
Fri				
Sat				

CALORIES TRACKER

Month: **Week of:**

	Breakfast	Lunch	Dinner	Snack
Sun				
Mon				
Tue				
Wed				
Thu				
Fri				
Sat				

CALORIES TRACKER

Month: **Week of:**

	Breakfast	Lunch	Dinner	Snack
Sun				
Mon				
Tue				
Wed				
Thu				
Fri				
Sat				

CALORIES TRACKER

Month: **Week of:**

	Breakfast	Lunch	Dinner	Snack
Sun				
Mon				
Tue				
Wed				
Thu				
Fri				
Sat				

CALORIES TRACKER

Month: **Week of:**

	Breakfast	Lunch	Dinner	Snack
Sun				
Mon				
Tue				
Wed				
Thu				
Fri				
Sat				

My Fitness Result Tracker

FITNESS RESULT

Starting Date: **Ending Date:**

Reminders

Before		After	
Chest		Chest	
Waist		Waist	
Hips		Hips	
Arm		Arm	
Thighs		Thighs	
Weight		Weight	
BMI		BMI	
Body Fat		Body Fat	
Muscle		Muscle	

Notes

FITNESS RESULT

Starting Date: **Ending Date:**

Reminders

Before		After	
Chest		Chest	
Waist		Waist	
Hips		Hips	
Arm		Arm	
Thighs		Thighs	
Weight		Weight	
BMI		BMI	
Body Fat		Body Fat	
Muscle		Muscle	

Notes

FITNESS RESULT

Starting Date: **Ending Date:**

Reminders	

Before		After	
Chest		Chest	
Waist		Waist	
Hips		Hips	
Arm		Arm	
Thighs		Thighs	
Weight		Weight	
BMI		BMI	
Body Fat		Body Fat	
Muscle		Muscle	

Notes

FITNESS RESULT

Starting Date: **Ending Date:**

Reminders

Before		After	
Chest		Chest	
Waist		Waist	
Hips		Hips	
Arm		Arm	
Thighs		Thighs	
Weight		Weight	
BMI		BMI	
Body Fat		Body Fat	
Muscle		Muscle	

Notes

FITNESS RESULT

Starting Date: **Ending Date:**

Reminders

Before		After	
Chest		Chest	
Waist		Waist	
Hips		Hips	
Arm		Arm	
Thighs		Thighs	
Weight		Weight	
BMI		BMI	
Body Fat		Body Fat	
Muscle		Muscle	

Notes

FITNESS RESULT

Starting Date: **Ending Date:**

Reminders

Before		After	
Chest		Chest	
Waist		Waist	
Hips		Hips	
Arm		Arm	
Thighs		Thighs	
Weight		Weight	
BMI		BMI	
Body Fat		Body Fat	
Muscle		Muscle	

Notes

FITNESS RESULT

Starting Date: **Ending Date:**

Reminders

Before		After	
Chest		Chest	
Waist		Waist	
Hips		Hips	
Arm		Arm	
Thighs		Thighs	
Weight		Weight	
BMI		BMI	
Body Fat		Body Fat	
Muscle		Muscle	

Notes

FITNESS RESULT

Starting Date: **Ending Date:**

Reminders

Before		After	
Chest		Chest	
Waist		Waist	
Hips		Hips	
Arm		Arm	
Thighs		Thighs	
Weight		Weight	
BMI		BMI	
Body Fat		Body Fat	
Muscle		Muscle	

Notes

FITNESS RESULT

Starting Date: **Ending Date:**

Reminders

Before		After	
Chest		Chest	
Waist		Waist	
Hips		Hips	
Arm		Arm	
Thighs		Thighs	
Weight		Weight	
BMI		BMI	
Body Fat		Body Fat	
Muscle		Muscle	

Notes

FITNESS RESULT

Starting Date: **Ending Date:**

Reminders

Before		After	
Chest		Chest	
Waist		Waist	
Hips		Hips	
Arm		Arm	
Thighs		Thighs	
Weight		Weight	
BMI		BMI	
Body Fat		Body Fat	
Muscle		Muscle	

Notes

FITNESS RESULT

Starting Date: **Ending Date:**

Reminders

Before		After	
Chest		Chest	
Waist		Waist	
Hips		Hips	
Arm		Arm	
Thighs		Thighs	
Weight		Weight	
BMI		BMI	
Body Fat		Body Fat	
Muscle		Muscle	

Notes

FITNESS RESULT

Starting Date: **Ending Date:**

Reminders

Before		After	
Chest		Chest	
Waist		Waist	
Hips		Hips	
Arm		Arm	
Thighs		Thighs	
Weight		Weight	
BMI		BMI	
Body Fat		Body Fat	
Muscle		Muscle	

Notes

FITNESS RESULT

Starting Date: **Ending Date:**

Reminders

Before		After	
Chest		Chest	
Waist		Waist	
Hips		Hips	
Arm		Arm	
Thighs		Thighs	
Weight		Weight	
BMI		BMI	
Body Fat		Body Fat	
Muscle		Muscle	

Notes

FITNESS RESULT

Starting Date: **Ending Date:**

Reminders

Before		After	
Chest		Chest	
Waist		Waist	
Hips		Hips	
Arm		Arm	
Thighs		Thighs	
Weight		Weight	
BMI		BMI	
Body Fat		Body Fat	
Muscle		Muscle	

Notes

FITNESS RESULT

Starting Date: **Ending Date:**

Reminders

Before		After	
Chest		Chest	
Waist		Waist	
Hips		Hips	
Arm		Arm	
Thighs		Thighs	
Weight		Weight	
BMI		BMI	
Body Fat		Body Fat	
Muscle		Muscle	

Notes

FITNESS RESULT

Starting Date: **Ending Date:**

Reminders

Before		After	
Chest		Chest	
Waist		Waist	
Hips		Hips	
Arm		Arm	
Thighs		Thighs	
Weight		Weight	
BMI		BMI	
Body Fat		Body Fat	
Muscle		Muscle	

Notes

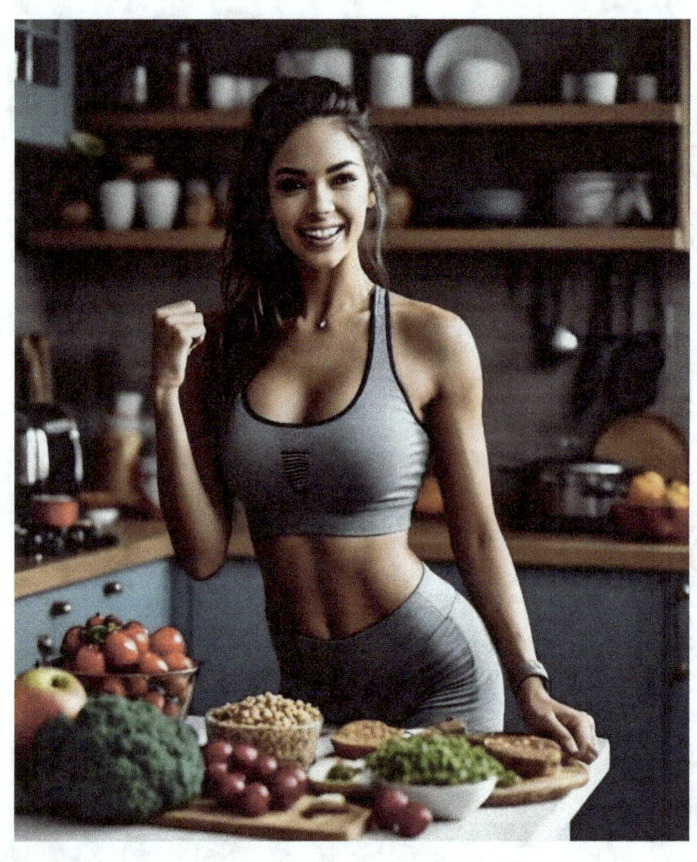